The Dangers of Diet Drugs and Other Weight-Loss Products

The Dangers of Diet Drugs and Other Weight-Loss Products

CeCe Barrett

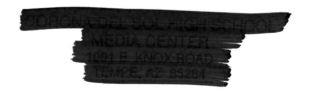

The Rosen Publishing Group/New York

The Teen Health
Library of
Eating Disorder
Prevention

I am indebted to Kathryn Nesbit, librarian at the Medical School of the University of Rochester, New York, for research materials on prescription diet drugs.

Published in 1999 by The Rosen Publishing Group, Inc.
29 East 21st Street, New York, NY 10010

Library of Congress Cataloging-in-Publication Data

Barrett, Cece.
  The dangers of diet drugs and other weight-loss products / Cece Barrett. — 1st ed.
          p.   cm. — (The Teen health library of eating disorder prevention)
  Includes index.
  Summary: Discusses the use of over-the-counter, prescription, and herbal diet drugs as well as liquid and prepackaged diet foods and explains their relation to eating disorders and proper nutrition.
  ISBN 1-8239-2768-7
  1. Appetite depressants—Health aspects—Juvenile literature. 2. Weight loss preparations—Health aspects—Juvenile literature. 3. Eating disorders—Juvenile literature. [1. Appetite depressants. 2. Weight loss preparations. 3. Eating disorders.]
    I. Title. II. Series.
  RM332.3.B37 1998S
  615'.73—dc21
                                                               98-29712
                                                                  CIP
                                                                  AC

Manufactured in the United States of America

Contents

Introduction

Michele wrote in her journal, "I'm still too fat." She underlined the words "too fat."

She got up from her chair and bent down to the bottom shelf of her bookcase. Removing the dictionary, she took out the bottle of diet pills she'd hidden behind it. Her friend Nadya had told her the pills would help her lose weight.

Michele was nervous as she opened the bottle and poured the shiny, red pills onto a tissue. But she was also desperate to lose weight. She popped one into her mouth.

After taking the pills for a few weeks, Michele didn't notice any weight loss, but she was having trouble sleeping, her hands trembled, her heart was constantly racing, and she was exhausted. Michele knew the diet pills were making her feel this way. She seemed to feel worse every day. She finally decided to stop taking the pills. Michele realized that losing a few pounds wasn't worth feeling so bad.

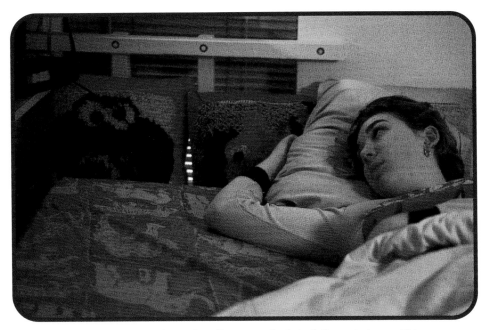

Using diet drugs may adversely affect your body's delicate balance. This can jeopardize your ability to relax and fall asleep at night and can affect your mood as well as your performance at school.

Michele's story shows the lengths to which some people will go in their efforts to lose weight. We live in a society that is obsessed with weight, body shape, fitness, and dieting. Our culture often sends out messages that you have to be thin in order to be desirable and successful. These messages can be seen everywhere—on television, in magazines and advertisements, and in the movies. The media encourage people to believe that they must be thin to be accepted by others. In response to these messages, many people go on diets to try to achieve a physical body shape that is often impossible for the average American to reach.

Millions of people in the United States are trying to lose weight every day. The weight-loss business is booming. An estimated $30 billion is spent on diet drugs and other weight-loss products in a year. A wide variety of products are on the market today that promise to help people shed their unwanted pounds.

Some products can be bought by anyone in local drugstores or health-food stores. Some drugs claim to be natural and safe aids to losing weight. Others are new and untested. There are also products that require a doctor's prescription. Nearly all are marketed with misleading or false claims about their powers and side effects. Some people also use products that are not meant for weight-loss purposes because they believe those products will help them lose weight.

What most people don't realize is that all these products can have dangerous, and even deadly, side effects. This book gives you honest, up-to-date information about the various products and methods that people often use in their quest to lose weight. You will learn the truth behind the claims and why using these products won't help anyone lose weight permanently.

This book will also discuss why so many people, both teens and adults, in this country are obsessed with their weight. Most important, you will learn why many experts believe that weight is not an important factor in being healthy and how the use of weight-loss products can lead to eating disorders and other problems.

Knowing the facts about the dangers of diet drugs will help you understand the importance of leading a healthy lifestyle—without diets or diet drugs. This book will also give you helpful suggestions on developing self-esteem and a positive body image, which are your best tools in preventing an eating disorder.

Over-the-Counter Diet Drugs

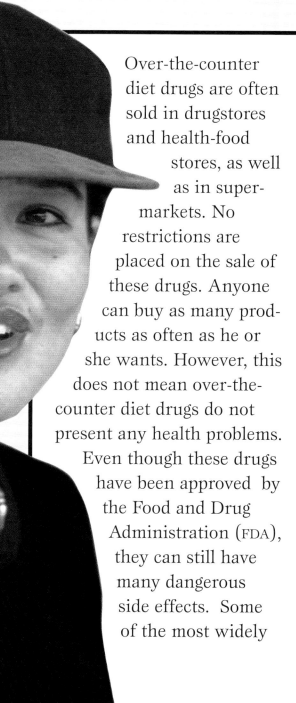

Over-the-counter diet drugs are often sold in drugstores and health-food stores, as well as in supermarkets. No restrictions are placed on the sale of these drugs. Anyone can buy as many products as often as he or she wants. However, this does not mean over-the-counter diet drugs do not present any health problems. Even though these drugs have been approved by the Food and Drug Administration (FDA), they can still have many dangerous side effects. Some of the most widely known over-the-counter diet drugs include Dexatrim, Acutrim, Thinz, and Appedrine.

If the drugs have been approved by the FDA, you may think that they are safe. But there have been many reports that question their safety. The main ingredient in all these over-the-counter drugs is called phenylpropanolamine, or PPA. PPA is a stimulant that resembles the illegal drugs known as amphetamines (speed). PPA can cause high blood pressure, anxiety, and nervousness. In addition to side effects, there is no proof that PPA helps people lose weight permanently. In fact, PPA has been banned in most countries.

In 1991, after a twenty-year investigation, the FDA came up with a list of more than 100 unsafe and ineffective ingredients used in over-the-counter diet aids. The whole point of the study was to stop companies from producing and selling diet products that didn't work and were dangerous to consumers. One ingredient that was not on the list was PPA.

Unfortunately, many drug companies have found ways to work around FDA regulations and ineffective products still find their way into the marketplace. In fact, according to Frances Berg, editor of the *Healthy Weight Journal*, Americans spend $5 billion to $7 billion a year on weight-loss products that don't work.

False Advertising

Some people who want to lose weight turn to diet pills because they believe the pills will help them become thinner. Many diet drug companies make false promises about the effectiveness of products. These products seem to provide easy and fast solutions to losing weight without exercising. In commercials and ads, the companies show before and after pictures of "real" people who have used their products. This sends the message that if you use their products, you too will become a slimmer and more attractive person in no time at all.

Sometimes it can be very

Diet drugs and other types of weight-loss products make many enticing promises and are easy to take. That's why some people mistakenly view them as an attractive alternative to a healthy diet and regular exercise.

hard not to believe these claims, and many people buy into the advertisements. It seems to be so easy to go to the drugstore around the corner, pick up a box of diet drugs, and immediately start losing weight.

But there are no such easy answers. If you read the fine print in the advertisements for these products, you will discover that the drugs will not help you lose weight permanently. Before you think about using an over-the-counter diet drug, it's important that you investigate the risks, as well as consider the reasons why you think you need to lose weight.

Labels

All manufacturers of diet drugs are required by the FDA to have a label that lists:

- ❏ the active ingredients in the drug
- ❏ any other ingredients
- ❏ the drug's intended purpose or purposes
- ❏ directions for use, including recom-
    mended dosages
- ❏ known side effects
- ❏ groups put at risk by the drug

Diet drugs and other over-the-counter drugs cannot be sold without such a label. The label is supposed to protect the consumer, but it also protects the company manufacturing the drug. If the consumer does not follow directions, the drug company can deny any responsibility for harmful reactions.

Reading the Labels

Labels on diet drugs are sometimes hard to understand. Although all the information required by the FDA is on the back of the box, it is often printed in very small letters. The information may also be hard to detect because slogans and claims are often printed on the packages in big, bold letters that draw your attention away from other information. These are designed to boost sales of the product. They make the diet drug seem safe and effective.

The slogans on diet drugs are easy to read. It takes time and effort to read the information required by the FDA. Yet it's also important to know that many diet drug manufacturers try to work around FDA regulations and others just ignore them. The FDA is not always able to pursue all consumer complaints.

Don't fall for promises that sound too good to be true. You are putting a drug, a foreign substance, into your body. This drug can have serious effects on your body.

Tanya was feeling low. She didn't make the cheerleading squad at her junior high school. All summer, she had practiced the routines, hoping to lead the fall pep rallies. Tanya told herself she was a total failure

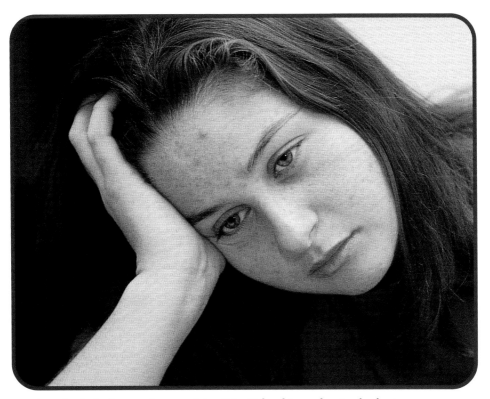

In today's body-conscious society, it isn't hard to understand why teens can easily become depressed over their appearance and turn to quick fixes, such as diet drugs, as a solution.

and that she didn't make the squad because she was too fat. She became more and more depressed.

Tanya decided she had to lose weight—fast. Skipping lunch and drinking diet cola wouldn't be enough. She decided to go to the drugstore after school the next day and buy some diet pills. When she went to the store, Tanya felt a little confused by all the choices. The one she picked said: "LOSE WEIGHT FAST."

When she got home, she told her mother that she had cramps and didn't feel up to eating dinner. She went to her room and took one of the pills. That night, she had trouble sleeping. When she got up the next morning, she *took two more pills. By noon she felt light-headed, but she didn't worry. She always felt extra nervous when she was dieting. By the end of the week, she was taking five or six pills at a time.*

Two weeks later, Tanya was taken to the emergency room of the local hospital. An overdose of the diet pills had caused heart failure. She was lucky. The doctors managed to save her life.

Why People Abuse Diet Drugs

Even though Tanya had read the instructions on the package, she still took more pills than the recommended dosage. Since she wanted to lose weight, she thought more pills would help her do that. And losing weight became more important than the possible side effects. Teens who are unhappy with their weight are especially vulnerable to over-the-counter diet drugs. Since the drugs are so easy and cheap to buy, many teens start to abuse them.

Also, because our culture places such importance on thinness, many people are willing to take serious risks in their efforts to lose weight. In one study conducted by Eating Disorders Awareness and Prevention (EDAP), researchers found that young girls are more afraid of becoming fat than they are of losing their parents, getting cancer, or nuclear war. And diet drug companies work hard to target those people who are most worried about their weight.

Physical Consequences

The medical journal *Pediatrics* compiled a list of negative side effects in young people who take over-the-counter diet drugs. These side effects are:

- ❏ seizures
- ❏ hallucinations
- ❏ confusion
- ❏ headaches
- ❏ mental disturbances
- ❏ anxiety
- ❏ paranoia
- ❏ mania
- ❏ hypertension
- ❏ cardiac irregularities

This report was given in 1990 during congressional hearings on diet pills led by Senator Ron Wyden of Oregon. The hearings were held in order to get the FDA to regulate PPA   so the drug

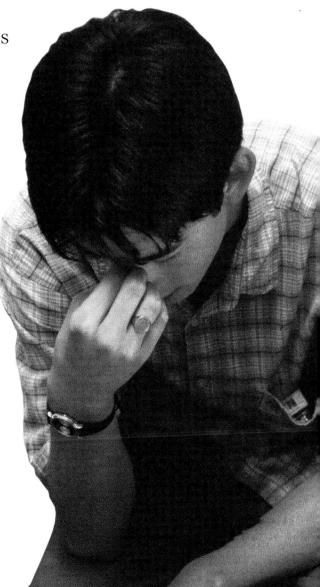

You might think that diet drugs will help you feel better about your body, but in reality they can cause you physical and mental pain.

would be available only by prescription. At the hearings, the president of the National Association of Anorexia Nervosa and Associated Disorders (ANAD) reported that teenagers with eating disorders often abuse diet pills. She said that in the last six years, there had been eleven reported cases of cerebral hemorrhage after taking PPA.

The FDA agreed to continue investigating PPA. Until further notice, the PPA-based drugs are still available to anyone who wants them.

Ipecac Syrup

Kaneesha wanted to be a model. At 5'7", 120 pounds, Kaneesha thought she had to lose weight to look like the models in all the fashion magazines that she read.

Kaneesha had two girlfriends who told her that vomiting was the best way to lose weight. They told her it was a great way to eat anything she wanted and not gain weight. Kaneesha didn't like the idea of sticking her fingers down her throat to make herself throw up. Then she found out about ipecac syrup. It was available at the drugstore. She drank the ipecac and threw up immediately.

At first, Kaneesha used ipecac syrup just once a week. Later, she used it two or three times a week, and sometimes more. She wasn't losing weight, her eyes were red, and she felt sick.

Kaneesha's worried mother took her to the doctor. After the doctor examined her, he asked her if she had ever used ipecac syrup. Kaneesha lied and said no. But the doctor knew that red eyes were the first sign of ipecac abuse and that Kaneesha could have died from using it.

Ipecac syrup is sometimes abused by people with bulimia nervosa, an eating disorder in which a person binges on a large amount of food and then purges it by vomiting.

Ipecac syrup is a powerful and extremely dangerous substance intended for emergency use only. If someone swallows poison, he or she is given a dose of ipecac syrup. Within a few minutes, he or she will throw up the poison. The vomiting induced by the syrup puts a tremendous strain upon the body. But because the person's life is in danger from the poison, it's worth the risk of taking ipecac syrup.

Because ipecac syrup has such dangerous consequences, it should be used only in emergency situations. Ipecac syrup can:

- become habit forming
- irritate the blood vessels around the eyes
- damage the digestive system
- damage heart tissue
- increase the risk of cardiac failure (death)

Laxatives
A laxative is a substance that causes bowel movements.

Laxatives can be bought over the counter in drugstores and grocery stores. Some teens use a laxative because they believe it will help the food they eat pass right through their bodies. But abusing laxatives can be very dangerous for many reasons. First, it dehydrates the body. When the body is dehydrated, it cannot function properly. It does not have enough water and it lacks the vital minerals contained in water.

Laxatives can also be addictive. If you use a laxative for more than a week, your body builds up a tolerance and you have to keep increasing the dosage in order for it to work. Eventually you can become addicted. Cramping, rectal bleeding, stomach pain, and dizziness are only some of the side effects of laxative abuse. It damages the intestines, the liver, and other vital organs.

Diuretics

Diuretics, or water pills, are another product used by some teens wishing to lose weight. Diuretics contain substances that speed up the action of the kidneys so that a person urinates more frequently. The formula varies from brand to brand. Some brands of water pills contain ammonium chloride, others contain caffeine.

Water pills reduce the amount of liquid in the body. A short-term loss of a pound or two may result. But the liquid and the weight come back very quickly.

The body responds to water pills by holding onto liquid. Water pills upset the normal functions of the body.

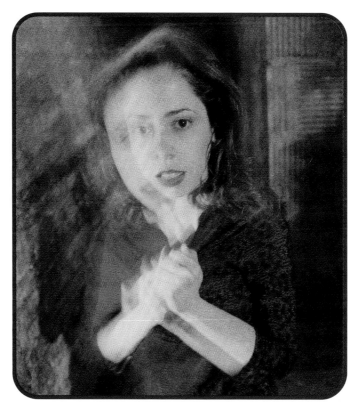

The use of prescription or over-the-counter diet drugs can cause you to feel dizzy or light-headed. You may also find yourself feeling stressed out and unable to relax.

So-called natural water pills are no better than chemically based diuretics. Both types put you at risk for dehydration and are habit forming.

The Bottom Line

Before you even consider taking an over-the-counter diet drug or any weight-loss product, think carefully about the consequences. In addition to the many side effects, diet drugs and other weight-loss products can lead a person to unhealthy weight management practices, or worse, a full-blown eating disorder.

Prescription Diet Drugs

2

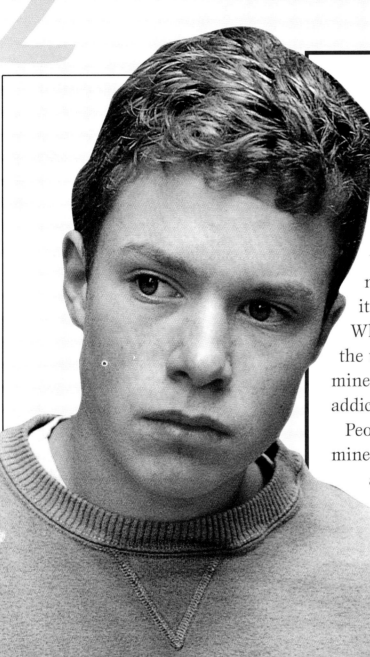

During the 1950s and 1960s, many doctors prescribed amphetamines to patients who wanted to lose weight.

Amphetamines speed up the body's central nervous system, causing it to burn more calories. What was not known at the time is that amphetamines are dangerous and addictive drugs.

People who took amphetamines lost weight, but many also developed an addiction to the drugs. The drugs increased the body's heart rate and blood pressure. This caused anxiety, nervousness, and insomnia. People then used other drugs, called depressants or downers, to slow down the body's functions. In many cases, the combination of these two types of drugs proved deadly. When the federal government and doctors realized the danger that amphetamines posed, restrictions were placed on their use.

Many of us believe that any drug prescribed by a physician is safe and helpful. Unfortunately, this is not always true. Prescription drugs can also have serious, sometimes deadly, effects on the body.

The Redux and Fen-phen Craze

In 1996, the FDA approved a new diet drug called dexfenfluramine, marketed under the name Redux™. It was thought by many to be the miracle diet pill. At the same time, a combination of drugs called fenfluramine and phentermine, or fen-phen, was being prescribed for weight loss. While the FDA had approved fenfluramine many years ago, it had not approved its combination with phentermine. Because fenfluramine was found to make people tired, drug manufacturers mixed it with phentermine, an amphetamine-like drug, to counteract the drowsiness.

Doctors have written a total of 18 million prescriptions for Redux and fen-phen. At the time the drugs were made available, scientists knew that the

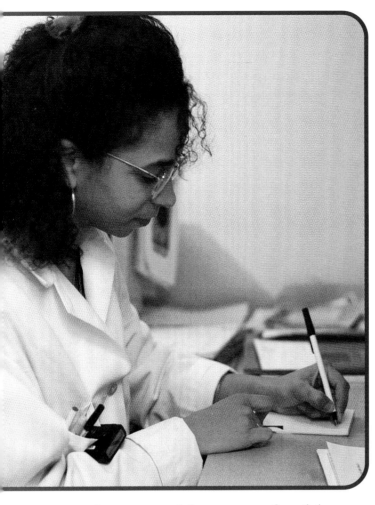

Scores of people received prescriptions for Redux and fen-phen from their doctors in the hope of losing weight quickly and effortlessly. Unfortunately, many doctors were unaware of the drugs' deadly side effects.

drugs could cause a fatal heart condition called pulmonary hypertension. But this condition is very rare, and many doctors believed that the risks of obesity outweighed the risks of the diet pills.

The active ingredients in Redux and fen-phen increase serotonin levels in the brain. Serotonin is a chemical that is basic to a person's emotional and physical sense of well-being. Scientists believe the mood-elevating effect of these drugs helps people to lose weight. Like other drugs, though,

Redux and fen-phen also caused side effects. Some of these effects are fatigue, diarrhea, and dry mouth. But over time, the drugs proved even more dangerous.

Diet Drugs and Weight-loss Centers

The danger of Redux and fen-phen increased partly because the drugs were supposed to be given to people under a doctor's supervision and only for short periods of time—no more than twelve weeks, according to the FDA. But many diet centers, such as Jenny Craig and Nutri/System, began making them available for unlimited periods of time. Redux and fen-phen were misused by many.

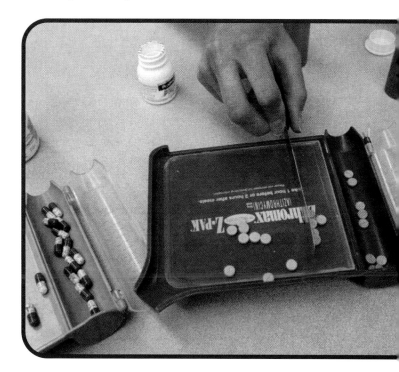

Many commercial weight-loss centers may have unknowingly contributed to the misuse of Redux and fen-phen by prescribing the drugs to clients for too long.

People who wanted to lose just a few pounds got prescriptions for Redux and fen-phen from their doctors or weight-loss clinics. But the problem was that many doctors who prescribed the drugs did not discuss their serious side effects with the patients. As a result, many people took the drugs without knowing about the drugs' dangers. And soon, other problems began to occur.

In 1997, Redux and fen-phen were taken off the market by the FDA. This was a very serious decision. Only twelve drugs have been recalled by the FDA in the past seventeen years. Many people had experienced dangerous effects from using these two drugs. Thirty percent of people who were taking the drugs suffered from heart valve damage. A number of people also died from using the two drugs. The drugs can cause the following side effects:

- insomnia
- memory loss
- depression
- abnormal heart rate
- damage to nerve endings
- permanent damage to the heart valves
- brain damage
- primary pulmonary hypertension (PPH), a disorder that can be deadly

More Prescription Drugs on the Way

The demand for diet drugs continues to be high because many people are willing to take the drugs despite their side effects. When Redux and fen-phen were taken off the market, people were waiting for something to take their place. They didn't have to wait long. Two months after Redux and fen-phen were recalled, the FDA approved a new drug called sibutramine hydrochloride monohydrate, which is marketed under the name Meridia.

According to an article in the *Los Angeles Times*, "Meridia can cause increases in blood pressure and, because it is believed to be psychologically and physically addictive, it is expected to be more tightly controlled and subject to regulation by the Drug Enforcement Administration." While this drug, too, was approved by the FDA, some doctors say they won't prescribe it because they believe the risks are too great. And ultimately, the real risks won't be known until the drug has been on the market for a while.

The Obesity Question

For years, doctors have said that obesity increases the risks of diabetes and heart disease and is the cause of more than 300,000 deaths each year in the United States. But these ideas about obesity are being questioned by many leading health experts.

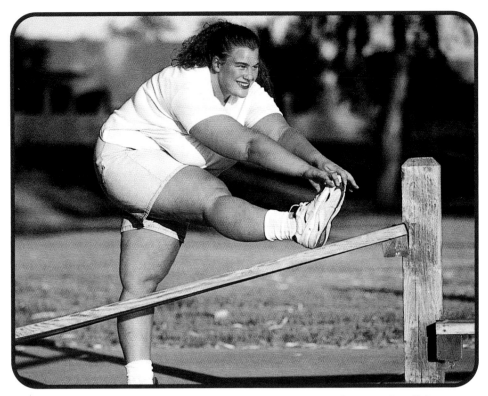

Regular exercise and healthy eating are more important indicators of well-being than how much a person weighs. It is possible for people with larger frames to carry additional weight without it necessarily posing a risk to their health.

According to David Levitsky, a nutrition and obesity expert at Cornell University, "Nobody ever dies of obesity." He believes that obesity is an indicator of other health problems that are caused by lack of exercise. Obesity alone is not a danger. "If you're a large person and you do not suffer from any other health problems, then there is no reason for you to lose weight."

Ultimately, it's more important to lead a healthy lifestyle and exercise regularly. Losing weight isn't always the answer. In fact, as Laura Fraser wrote in *Losing It: America's Obsession with Weight and the Industry that Feeds on It*: "Even if there are considerable health risks to severe obesity, there is no evidence that medical weight-loss treatments lessen those risks. There are, however, good indications that those treatments can lead to depression, eating disorders, physically stressful yo-yo dieting, and with some treatments, serious side effects and even death."

Herbal Diet Drugs

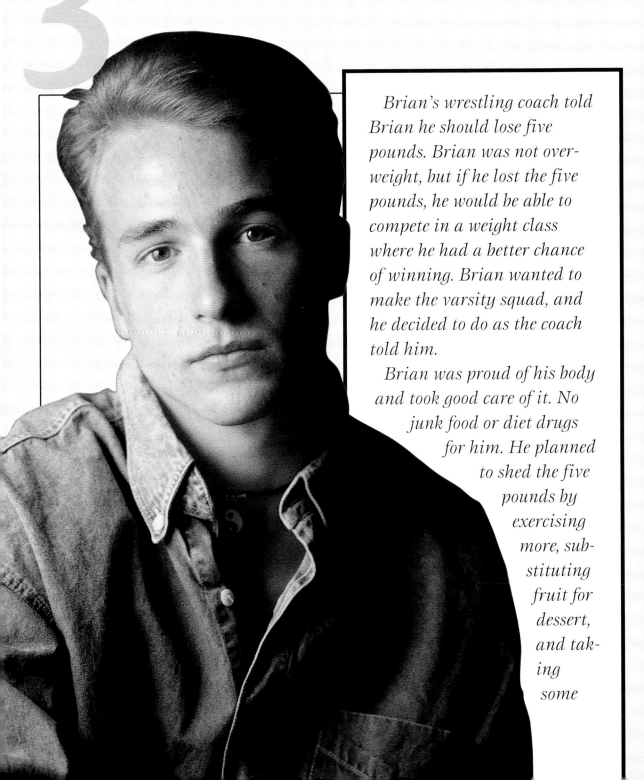

Brian's wrestling coach told Brian he should lose five pounds. Brian was not overweight, but if he lost the five pounds, he would be able to compete in a weight class where he had a better chance of winning. Brian wanted to make the varsity squad, and he decided to do as the coach told him.

Brian was proud of his body and took good care of it. No junk food or diet drugs for him. He planned to shed the five pounds by exercising more, substituting fruit for dessert, and taking some *herbal supplements. At the diet and fitness section of a nutrition store, Brian noticed a product with the slogan, "Nature's fen-phen." Since it contained nothing but herbs and was supposed to be a natural way to lose weight, Brian decided to give it a try.*

The next day, Brian got up early and ran three miles. He took one of the herbal pills with breakfast. He figured he would see how the pills made him feel before he took any more. About an hour later, he noticed that his heart and his thoughts were racing. By the time he got to wrestling practice, he hardly knew what he was doing. Brian started yelling and cursing at the coach. Then, all of a sudden, he burst into tears.

In recent years, more and more people in the United States have started buying products labeled "natural." Many people mistakenly believe that anything natural is healthy or safe. But some natural substances can be just as harmful and as strong as prescription drugs. Others need to be used with caution. Some herbal remedies have been used for medicinal purposes in various countries for many years. Taken properly, some may be helpful in relieving certain ailments, but most herbal products have not been subjected to any kind of testing, and there is often no way to determine whether or not they are safe.

Currently, many herbal diet drugs are on the market. Pharmacies may stock some of them, but specialty

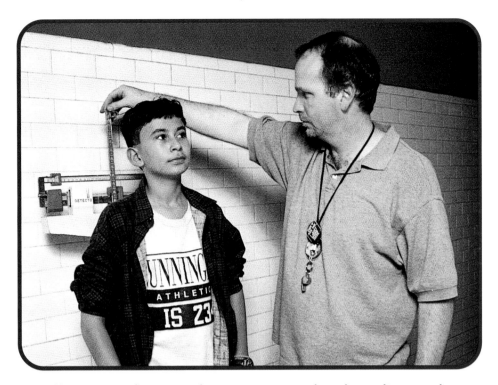

Different types of sports, such as gymnastics, track, and wrestling, can place additional pressure on participants if they are expected to maintain a certain weight or have a specific type of physical build.

stores, such as nutrition stores or vitamin stores, are the main suppliers. Right now, herbal diet drugs are the best-selling weight-loss products on the U.S. market. People started buying them as an alternative to the prescription diet drugs that had been recalled by the FDA. Many believe herbal diet drugs are safer than those made from chemicals because herbs are natural.

Nature's Fen-phen

One of the most popular herbal diet drugs on the market today is known as herbal fen-phen. The name is a sneaky way of linking herbal fen-phen to the prescription drug fen-phen. The manufacturers want consumers to think that herbal fen-phen is as effective as prescription fen-phen, but without the dangerous side effects because their version of fen-phen is natural.

One of the key ingredients in herbal fen-phen is St.-John's-wort. St.-John's-wort is an herb that lifts people's moods, but it can also make them extremely sensitive to sunlight. St.-John's-wort can be especially harmful to those with fair skin.

The other key ingredient in this herbal diet drug is called either ma huang or ephedra. This ingredient speeds up the central nervous system, which supposedly can help people burn more calories. But ephedra can also be addictive and have dangerous consequences. In one year alone, thirty-eight deaths have been attributed to heart failure caused by ephedra-based products.

Ephedra-based products were being used for getting high as an alternative to illegal street drugs. This caused the FDA to issue warnings about the products. Many states have banned the sale of ephedra-based drugs to minors. But the same drugs are still available to minors in other products that claim to aid in weight loss.

Herbal Dieter's Tea

There are many herbal teas on the market that claim to help people lose weight. But they, too, have serious side effects. The main ingredient in most of these teas is an herb called senna. Senna works as a laxative and it can cause diarrhea and cramping. If used for a long time senna depletes the body of potassium, which can cause problems with the heart and colon. Without potassium, the heart beats irregularly. Heart-rhythm disturbances have resulted in many deaths. As a result of such deaths, the FDA recommended that many herbal diet teas carry labels warning that the teas contain laxatives and could cause serious side effects, and even death.

Energy Pills

Energy pills make no claims of helping a person to lose weight. Instead they claim to help a person stay with a diet and exercise program. Manufacturers make the assumption that dieting can make a person so weak and tired that he or she won't want to exercise, and will be more likely to eat a fattening snack. They claim that energy pills will give you energy. You will then be more likely to stick to your diet and exercise program.

But ask yourself: How do energy pills provide energy? Energy pills contain one or more of the following stimulants: ginseng, green tea, guarana, kola nut, yerba mate, ephedra, and sometimes caffeine. The energy that these substances provide isn't the kind you get from eating healthy foods and exercising regularly. Rather, these substances create a kind of energy that can make you feel anxious and jittery.

The FDA and Herbal Products

Another important factor to keep in mind is that the FDA has little control over the sale of herbs. In 1994, the U.S. Congress passed the Dietary Supplement Health and Education Act. This act made it legal to sell so-called natural substances over the counter without FDA testing. Companies have the right to sell herbs, vitamins, and minerals without testing them to see if they are safe and effective. The only restriction the FDA imposes is to limit the claims that a manufacturer can make for a product. For example, a product cannot claim to cure illness, but it can say how the product affects the body.

The end result is a variety of untested products on the market. Without FDA control of the sale of these products, a consumer cannot tell whether they are safe or effective.

Liquid Meals and Other Weight-Loss Products

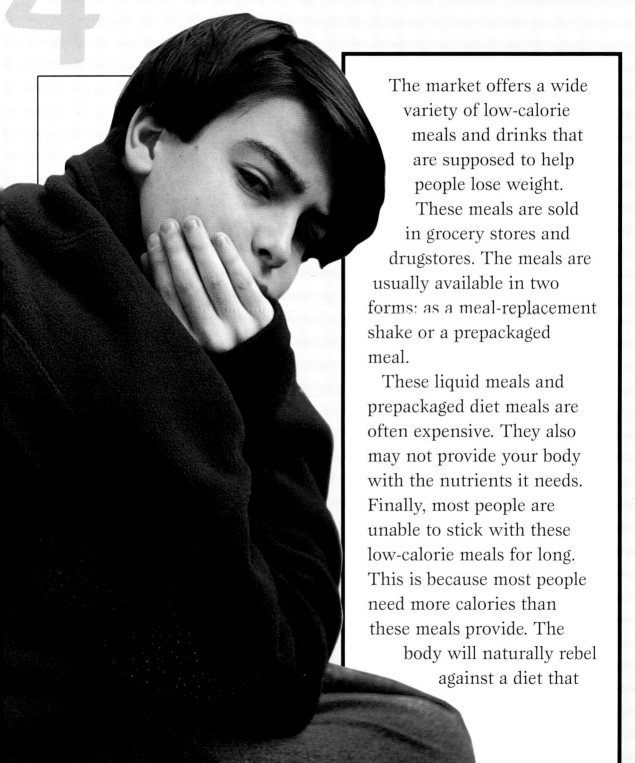

The market offers a wide variety of low-calorie meals and drinks that are supposed to help people lose weight. These meals are sold in grocery stores and drugstores. The meals are usually available in two forms: as a meal-replacement shake or a prepackaged meal.

These liquid meals and prepackaged diet meals are often expensive. They also may not provide your body with the nutrients it needs. Finally, most people are unable to stick with these low-calorie meals for long. This is because most people need more calories than these meals provide. The body will naturally rebel against a diet that doesn't give the body what it needs. Any weight that is lost often returns after people stop eating the low-calorie meals.

Liquid Meals

Kyra was watching television when a commercial came on. A young woman was talking about a meal-replacement shake that helped her lose five pounds in five days. Kyra thought the diet shakes were a great way to lose weight. The drink she saw on the television ad looked like a chocolate shake.

The next day, Kyra went to the drugstore and bought a package of the drink. The box included fifteen packages of shake mix and a five-day diet and exercise plan. During the five days, she was instructed to drink three shakes a day and eat nothing but fruits and vegetables.

Two days into the plan, Kyra was starving. Visions of pepperoni pizza, ice cream, and cookies floated through her mind. She became so hungry that when she got home from school on the third day, she ate practically everything in sight. She ate until she felt ill. Afterward, she was disgusted with herself. Not only had the liquid meals been a failure, but they had caused her to totally lose control over food.

One of the problems with liquid meals is that they cannot sustain a person for long. It's impossible for one shake to replace an entire meal and still provide

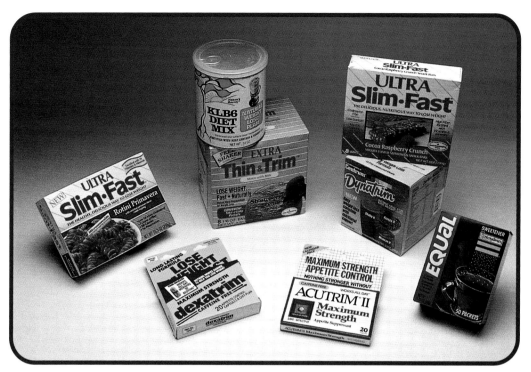

Over-the-counter diet drugs and weight-loss products cannot take the place of well-rounded, healthy meals that include fresh fruits and vegetables, grains, and natural sources of protein.

the body with the nutrients it needs. Although the package says the liquid diet offers lots of nutrients, the nutrients come from synthetic substances. Synthetic substances cannot give the body the nourishment it needs to develop. This is especially true for teens whose bodies are still growing and developing. The body needs food to fuel its processes.

One brand of liquid meals claims to provide vitamin A, vitamin C, iron, calcium, and many more healthful substances. This sounds good until you read the list of ingredients: sugar, fructose, dextrose, cornstarch, cellulose gel, cupric sulfate, and other chemicals. If you continue reading the label, you learn that skim milk powder is the main source of the vitamins and minerals in the product.

The body needs a certain amount of calories to carry out daily bodily functions. When it doesn't receive the fuel it needs, the results are fatigue and lack of energy. A person may also feel weak or light-headed.

Prepackaged Diet Meals

Two types of prepackaged diet meals are generally available. One kind can be purchased at most grocery stores. The other kind is available only if you join a weight-loss program, such as Jenny Craig or Nutri/System.

Prepackaged diet meals are low in calories, just like the liquid diet shakes. If you purchase them through a weight-loss program, it can be very expensive. Not only do you have to pay for the costs of the meals, you also need to pay a membership fee to join the program.

People have the same problems with diet meals that they do with diet drinks. It's difficult to stay on a diet that continually deprives the body of the calories and nutrients it needs.

Recent research indicates that fresh food is healthier and more flavorful than prepackaged food. Once food is frozen or canned, it loses valuable vitamins and minerals. Preservatives are chemicals that are

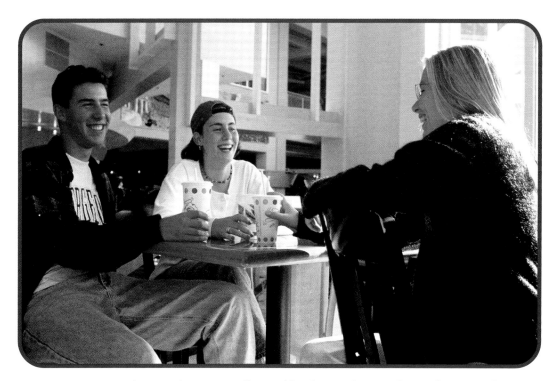

Your attitude toward eating is influenced by the people around you. If you spend time with friends who have positive attitudes toward food, it may improve how you feel about eating.

added to keep food from spoiling. Because preservatives are chemicals, they should not be part of every meal.

Think About It

One important point that is often overlooked in the discussion of diet pills and weight-loss products is money. The makers of diet pills and weight-loss products are in business to make a profit. In order to do that, they must create a need for their products. The best way to create a need for weight-loss products is to convince consumers that being overweight is unhealthy and unattractive. If you actually liked your body and accepted yourself at whatever size you happen to be, you would have no need for these products—and then perhaps those companies wouldn't have so many customers.

Ultimately, it's not in the company's best interest for you to like who you are. But it's in your best interest to accept yourself and your body. It's your best defense in the fight against eating disorders.

Diet Drugs and Eating Disorders

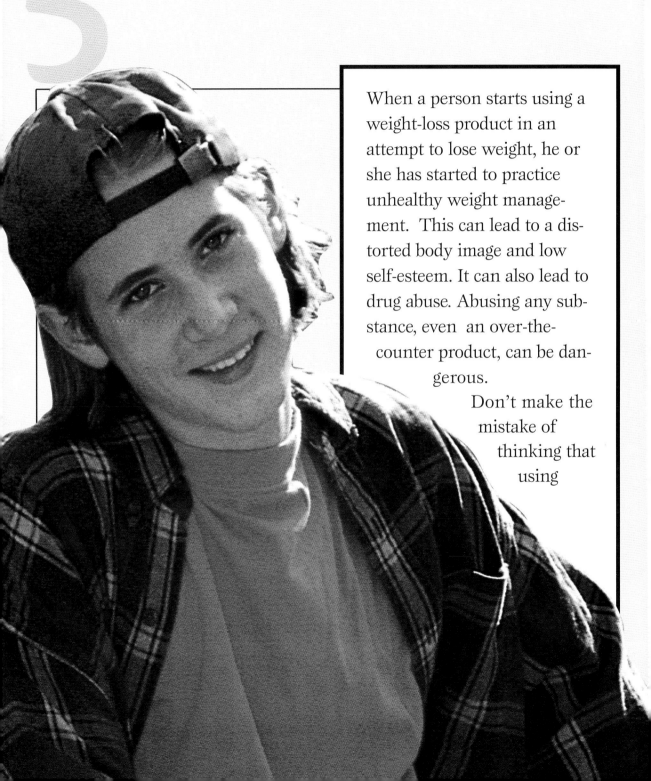

When a person starts using a weight-loss product in an attempt to lose weight, he or she has started to practice unhealthy weight management. This can lead to a distorted body image and low self-esteem. It can also lead to drug abuse. Abusing any substance, even an over-the-counter product, can be dangerous.

Don't make the mistake of thinking that using

caffeine, ipecac syrup, or other weight-loss products is a minor matter. If you are abusing diet pills or other weight-loss products, it's important that you speak with someone about your problem. A parent, an older sibling, your doctor, or a teacher can help you get the help you need.

There are many physical and emotional consequences related to using/abusing diet drugs and other weight-loss products. While we have already discussed the physical reactions to most of these products, the mind also suffers greatly when a person goes on a diet. In this chapter, you will learn what happens when a person goes on a diet and why diets do not work. We will also discuss how the use of diet products can lead to the development of an eating disorder, and how to recognize if you have a problem.

Diets Do Not Work

The body needs a certain amount of calories every day. The food we eat is converted into fuel for the body to carry on its normal processes. When we do not provide the body with this necessary fuel, it tries to conserve fuel to survive by slowing down its metabolism, or the rate at which the body burns calories. When this metabolic rate is lowered, the body burns fewer calories and stores fat more efficiently.

When you eat less, your body responds by holding on to any food it gets. When a person goes off the

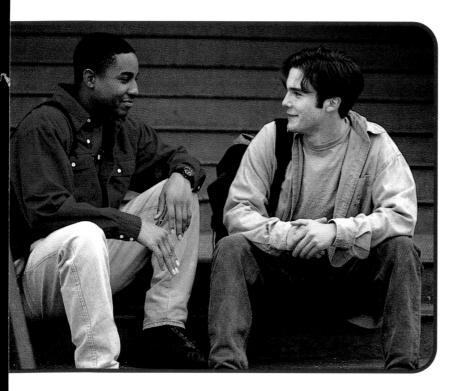

Your teen years are a demanding time. Taking over-the-counter or prescription diet drugs can have negative effects on both your mental and physical well-being.

diet, the body will regain all of the weight lost during the diet, if not more. This is because the metabolism does not return to normal after a diet.

In addition to being ineffective, dieting can also physically damage the body. The teen years are a time of great mental and physical growth. During this period, the body is changing from a child's body into an adult's. The body needs fuel to make this transformation successfully. If it fails to receive this fuel, important bodily functions, such as a young woman's menstruation, may be delayed. A lack of nutrients can also lead to osteoporosis, a disease that weakens the bones.

Another danger of dieting is the attitude it can create. When a diet is unsuccessful, a person's self-esteem suffers. He or she may feel like a failure when weight is not lost permanently. He or she can begin an unhealthy cycle of yo-yo dieting. Yo-yo dieting is when a person begins and quits a diet several times. A person may focus all his or her attention on losing weight. He or she may begin to lose touch with reality and become desperate in the quest to lose weight. Taking diet pills or other weight-loss products is only the beginning of an unhealthy pattern of behavior. It is possible that this pattern may eventually lead to the development of an eating disorder.

Because of a greater awareness about the importance of proper nutrition, it has become easier to make smart and delicious choices about the foods you eat. Vegetable juices, fruit smoothies, and even skim milk are all popular ways to satisfy hunger in a healthy way.

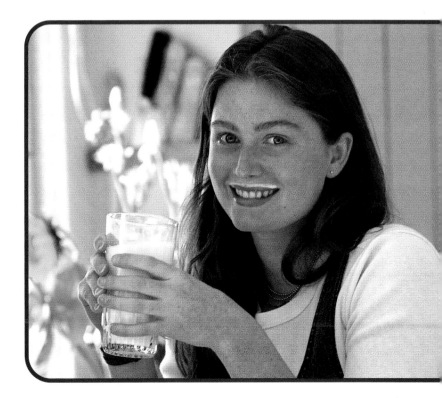

What Is an Eating Disorder?

Eating disorders include anorexia nervosa, bulimia nervosa, and binge-eating disorder (compulsive eating). Compulsive exercise is also a growing problem and is classified by experts as an eating disorder–related problem. A person can have one or more of these disorders, and anyone can suffer from them—men and women of all ages and ethnic backgrounds.

According to studies, 80 percent of people with anorexia nervosa or bulimia nervosa began their bout with these disorders after going on a diet. Almost eight million people in the United States have eating disorders. While most eating disorders affect females, an increasing number of males are developing them. An eating disorder is extremely dangerous—physically and mentally. If it is not treated properly, it can lead to permanent damage and even death.

People with anorexia nervosa intentionally starve themselves to lose weight. The problem is that no matter how much weight is lost, people with anorexia never think it is enough. Anorexia causes people to see their bodies in a distorted manner. People with anorexia may be of average weight or even below average weight, but they believe they are too fat and need to lose more weight.

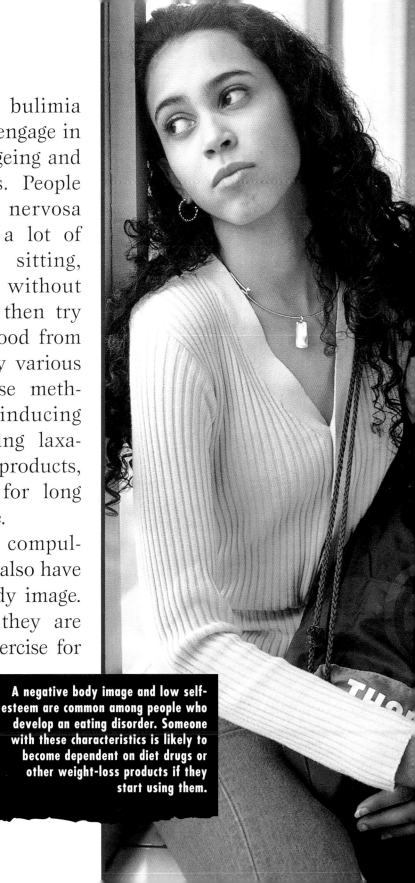

People with bulimia nervosa often engage in unhealthy bingeing and purging cycles. People with bulimia nervosa binge, or eat a lot of food in one sitting, often eating without control. They then try to purge the food from their bodies by various methods. These methods include inducing vomiting, taking laxatives or other products, or exercising for long periods of time.

People who compulsively exercise also have a distorted body image. They believe they are fat and will exercise for hours at a time every day, often secretly, so they

A negative body image and low self-esteem are common among people who develop an eating disorder. Someone with these characteristics is likely to become dependent on diet drugs or other weight-loss products if they start using them.

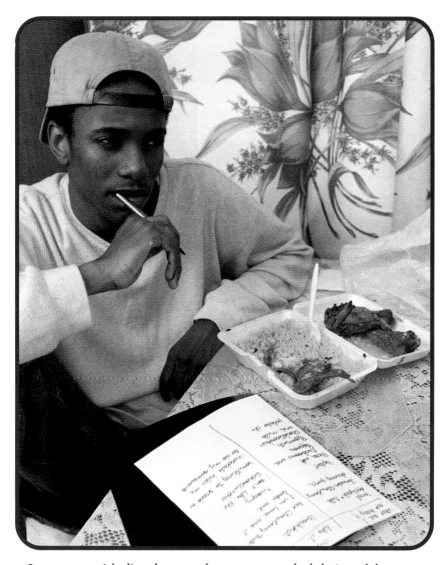

Because teens' bodies change and grow a great deal during adolescence, poor eating habits or an eating disorder can be especially harmful to young people's development.

will continue to lose weight. They may also force themselves to vomit or abuse diet pills and/or laxatives.

People who eat compulsively often use food as a way to cope with problems in their lives. They have an unhealthy relationship with food, and they need help to deal with their problems. Unlike other eating disorders, people suffering from compulsive eating are not trying to lose weight. These people may eat large amounts of food, but they will not try to rid the body of the food.

It's important to note that the symptoms of these eating disorders are interchangeable. This means a person with bulimia may also try to starve him- or herself, and a person with anorexia may also exercise compulsively.

Eating Disorder Warning Signs

Some common signs of an eating disorder are:

- ❐ constantly thinking about the size and shape of your body
- ❐ constantly thinking about how much you weigh and weighing yourself repeatedly during the day
- ❐ constantly thinking about food, cooking, and eating
- ❐ eating only certain foods in specific and limited amounts
- ❐ keeping a list of what foods are okay to eat
- ❐ wanting to eat alone and feeling uncomfortable eating with other people
- ❐ not feeling good about yourself unless you are thin, but never being satisfied

with how thin you are
- ❑ thinking that you should exercise more, no matter how much you do exercise
- ❑ feeling competitive about dieting and wanting to be the thinnest or the smallest
- ❑ taking diet pills or laxatives
- ❑ continuing to diet, even after you are thin
- ❑ purposely losing lots of weight very quickly
- ❑ forcing yourself to throw up
- ❑ no longer having your monthly period

If anything on this list describes you, you may have an eating disorder. You don't have to have every symptom on the list to have an eating disorder. If some of these sound familiar, please consider getting help.

Dangers of Eating Disorders

Eating disorders are a serious matter. They can permanently damage your body. A person can also die from an eating disorder. Even with professional help, it takes a long time to recover from an eating disorder, but many people do recover and go on to live successful, healthy lives.

If you think you may be suffering from one or

more of these eating disorders, it's important that you reach out for help. Talk to someone you trust and seek professional help. There is a list of organizations in the Where to Go for Help section at the back of this book. You can contact one or more of them for more information and resources in your area. With the proper help, you can begin to recover from the disorder and take back control of your life.

Taking Care of Yourself

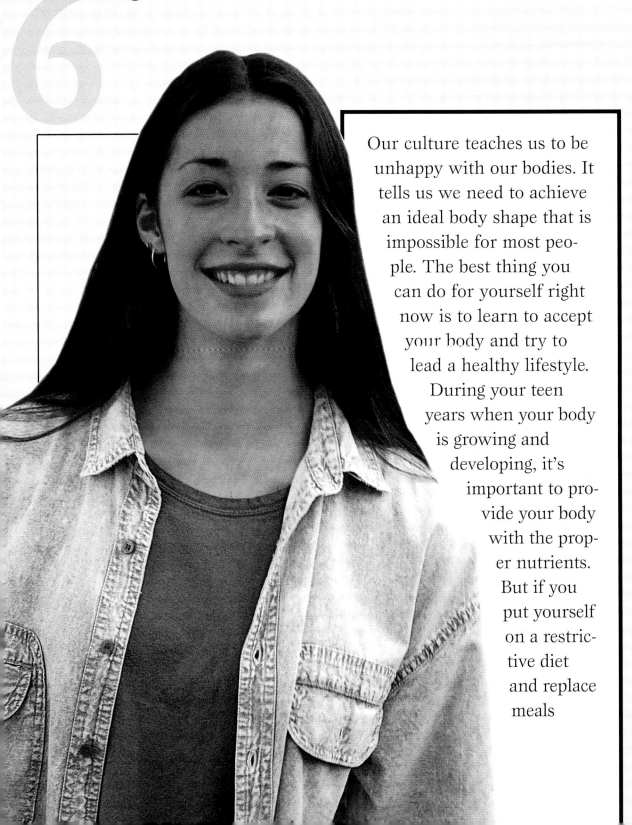

Our culture teaches us to be unhappy with our bodies. It tells us we need to achieve an ideal body shape that is impossible for most people. The best thing you can do for yourself right now is to learn to accept your body and try to lead a healthy lifestyle. During your teen years when your body is growing and developing, it's important to provide your body with the proper nutrients. But if you put yourself on a restrictive diet and replace meals with diet pills and other weight-loss products, you are depriving your body of the nutrients it needs to grow and develop properly. Not only does dieting hurt your body, but it is also ineffective. It can lead to other serious conditions, such as an eating disorder or addiction to substances that you believe help you lose weight.

Ask yourself why you want to lose weight. Do you think you will be happier or healthier if you lose weight? If you do, it's important to recognize that many leading health experts now question the importance of weight. Being healthy involves much more than a number on a scale. Being healthy means eating well and exercising regularly. It's also important to remember that your worth as a person is not connected with your weight.

Accept Your Body

Each person is born with genes that determine how he or she will look physically, from the color of the eyes, to height, to the type of body he or she will have. These are qualities that make each of us unique. No matter how hard some people may try or what kind of diet they go on, they will never look like a supermodel.

Many teens often fall into the trap of comparing themselves to the beautiful, thin people in movies, television, and advertisements. Some teens believe the people they see in the media are the norm. But if you take a look around at the people in your life—your friends, family, classmates, and even the people you see on the street—you'll realize that there are many different body types and many different kinds of beauty. You'll also notice that not many people look like the people in the movies or ads.

No one is perfect. This includes the people you see in the media. We all have qualities that make each of us unique and special. This is why you should never compare yourself to another person. You have unique qualities that no one else has. Learn to accept yourself—emotionally and physically.

Improve Your Body Image

One of the best ways to avoid comparing yourself to others is to build your self-confidence. Have faith in your abilities and yourself. When you feel good about and believe in yourself, you are less likely to be tempted to try to change yourself. Confidence is the foundation of good mental and physical health. The next time you start putting yourself down, stop and tell yourself:

> ❐ I will remember that being thin does not make me a happier person.
> ❐ I will stop comparing my body with other people's bodies.
> ❐ I will exercise because it's fun, not because it burns calories.

❏ I will do things that make me feel good about myself and that don't revolve around my body shape and size.
❏ I will value other people for who they are, not what they look like.

Exercise and Eat Right

Eating nutritious foods and exercising regularly will go a long way to improve the quality of your life. While you now know that dieting is unhealthy, it does not mean that you shouldn't think about what you eat.

Eating well-balanced meals of lean meats, fruits and vegetables, milk and other dairy products, and grains is an important part of healthy eating. While it's important to avoid too much sugar, salt, or caffeine, healthy eating does not mean that you have to completely deprive yourself. We all have busy lives, and we cannot eat sensibly all the time. There will also be times when you crave a candy bar or french fries, and it's perfectly fine to give in to the craving occasionally. The secret is moderation. Keep your meals balanced. Always make your health a priority, not a number on a scale or the size of your clothes.When you don't routinely deny yourself the foods you want, you are more likely to eat well overall.

Exercise is also an important part of staying fit and healthy. It is recommended that a person exercise

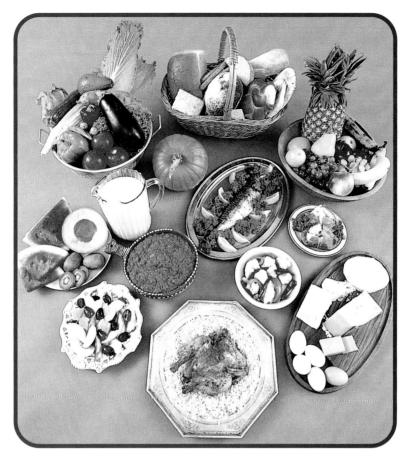

Teens have so many delicious and nutritious foods from which to choose that they should never need diet drugs or any weight-loss products to stay healthy and fit.

for thirty minutes or more at least three times a week. This does not mean that you have to go to the gym every day and work out for hours at a time. You should make exercising into a fun activity. Go biking with a friend, try in-line skating, or go for a long walk. Join the school track team. Do anything that you find enjoyable and that gets you on your feet and gets your heart beating faster.

You should not think of exercise just as a way to lose weight. If you do, you may become frustrated when you fail to see the results you want. There are many benefits to exercise. It helps to strengthen your body. It increases your confidence in yourself and your body. It reduces stress and makes you feel good.

Speak Out Against Diet Culture

Even after you learn everything about the dangers of diet drugs, it's not easy to give up the idea of dieting and accept yourself at whatever size you happen to be. Every day, you may encounter images and messages from family, friends, and society that praise the thin and punish the fat. These ideas are hard to ignore. But you are not powerless against them. Speaking out against fat prejudice and diet culture is a great way to improve your own self-esteem and create awareness about the dangers of diets.

Create a support group at your school or among your friends. Write a letter to a television network or fashion magazine when you see images that you don't like. Talk to your parents and teachers about what you've learned in this book. All these things will help you develop a healthy self-image that will give you the confidence to keep a positive attitude about food and weight for the rest of your life.

Glossary

addict A person with a psychological and physical dependency on alcohol, a drug, or a behavior.

amino acids The chemical building blocks of proteins, which are essential to life.

anorexia nervosa An eating disorder in which a person refuses to eat and keeps losing weight.

appetite suppressant A drug that is supposed to control hunger.

binge-eating disorder (compulsive eating) An eating disorder in which a person eats large amounts of food but does not purge.

bulimia nervosa An eating disorder in which a person eats large amounts of food and then gets rid of it by purging.

caffeine A chemical substance, often found in tea or coffee, that stimulates the nervous system.

dehydration Excessive loss of water from the body.

depression   A condition in which a person feels sad for a long period of time and has trouble concentrating and sleeping.

diuretic (water pill)   A drug that causes an increase in the amount of urine put out by the kidneys.

ephedra (ma huang)   An herb that works as a stimulant and is found in many so-called natural diet drugs.

laxative   A substance that causes bowel movements.

prescription   A note from a doctor that allows a person to purchase a regulated drug.

psychologist   A health care professional trained to handle emotional and behavioral problems.

purge   To rid the body of food or calories.

serotonin   A chemical substance in the brain that regulates mood and appetite.

side effect   Undesirable secondary effect of a drug.

stimulant   An herb, drug, or other substance that activates the nervous system.

Where to Go for Help

American Anorexia/Bulimia Association (AABA)
165 West 46th Street
Suite 1108
New York, NY 10036
(212)575-6200
Web site: http://members.aol.com/AMANBU

Anorexia Nervosa and Related Eating Disorders, Inc. (ANRED)
P.O. Box 5102
Eugene, OR 97405
(541)344-1144
Web site: http://www.anred.com

Eating Disorders Awareness and Prevention, Inc. (EDAP)
603 Stewart Street, Suite 803
Seattle, WA 98101
(206) 382-3587
Web site: http://members.aol.com/edapinc

National Association of Anorexia Nervosa and Associated Disorders (ANAD)
P.O. Box 7
Highland Park, IL 60035
(847)831-3438
Web site:
http://members.aol.com/anad20/index.html

Overeaters Anonymous (OA)
P.O. Box 44020
Rio Rancho, NM 87174-4020
(505)891-2664
Web site: http://www.overeatersanonymous.org

In Canada

Anorexia Nervosa and Associated Disorders (ANAD)
109-2040 West 12th Avenue
Vancouver, BC V6J 2G2
(604) 739-2070

The National Eating Disorder Information Centre
College Wing, 1st floor, Room 211
200 Elizabeth Street
Toronto, ON M5G 2C4
(416) 340-4156

For Further Reading

Adderholdt-Elliott, Miriam. *Perfectionism: What's Bad About Being Too Good?* Minneapolis, MN: Free Spirit Publishers, 1987.

Cooke, Kaz. *Real Gorgeous: The Truth About Body and Beauty.* New York: W.W. Norton, 1996.

Fraser, Laura. *Losing It: America's Obsession with Weight and the Industry that Feeds on It.* New York: Dutton, 1997.

Hall, Liza F. *Perk! The Story of a Teenager with Bulimia.* Carlsbad, CA: Gürze Books, 1997.

Hesse-Biber, Sharlene. *Am I Thin Enough Yet?* Oxford: Oxford University Press, 1996.

Kolodny, Nancy J. *When Food's a Foe: How You Can Confront and Conquer Your Eating Disorder.* Boston: Little Brown and Company, 1992.

Kubersky, Rachel. *Everything You Need to Know About Eating Disorders: Anorexia and Bulimia.* Rev. ed. New York: The Rosen Publishing Group, 1998.

Pipher, Mary. *Hunger Pains.* New York: Ballantine Books, 1997.

Index

About the Author

CeCe Barrett is a writer and teacher who lives in New York City. She earned a B.A. from Vassar College and a Ph.D. from Yale University. She is married and has two teenage daughters.

Design and Layout: Christine Innamorato

Consulting Editor: Michele I. Drohan

Photo Credits

Photo on p. 7 by Kathleen McClancy; pp. 10, 47 by Telegraph Colour Library/FPG International; p. 12 by Ira Fox; pp. 15, 17 by Ethan Zindler; pp. 21, 32 by John Bentham; p. 22 by Jill Sabella/FPG International; p. 24 by Seth Dinnerman; p. 25 by PhotoDisc; p. 28 by Ken Ross/FPG International; pp. 30, 36, 44 by Ron Chapple/FPG International; p. 38 by Jonathan Meyers/FPG International; p. 40 by Mark Harmel/FPG International; p. 42 by Steven Jones/FPG International; p. 45 by Stephen Simpson/FPG International; p. 48 by Maike Schulz; p. 52 by Scott Brown/International Stock; p. 56 byFrank Siteman/Viesti Associates, Inc.